Palliative Care
and
Euthanasia

Palliative Care
and
Euthanasia

Edited by
Frank A Huser

with papers by
Elizabeth G Jones, Maureen McLellan,
Janice Turner, Susan A Hodge, Janny A Teule,
Leonard J van der Hout,
and Gusta van den Bogaard

Campion Press, Edinburgh
1995

British Library Cataloguing in Publication Data:

Palliative Care and Euthanasia
1. Huser, Frank A.
610.7361

ISBN 1 873732 16 3

The publishers are grateful for the co-operation of

— **North East Surrey College of Technology
Faculty of Humanities, Health and Nursing
Epsom, England**

and

**Christelijke Hogeschool Windesheim
Institute for Higher Education
Faculty of Health Care
Zwolle, The Netherlands**

© **1995 Campion Press**

Published by Campion Press
384 Lanark Road, Edinburgh EH13 0LX

Designed and typeset in 10/12pt Palatino by Artisan Graphics, Edinburgh
Printed and bound by Bell and Bain, Glasgow

Preface

During the last few years, public awareness of the issues surrounding euthanasia has greatly increased and a great deal of debate has ensued. The subject is inextricably linked with political and religious dogmas and doctrines, but nothing should obscure the fact that at the centre of the argument lie real and painful questions of how best to care for the seriously and the terminally ill. Issues of death cannot be separated from those of life, and the processes of terminal care are in every sense care for the living.

In the autumn of 1993, a symposium on the theme 'Palliative Care and Euthanasia' was held in London, and the papers presented there have been collected into this book. They covered the legal, ethical and socio-logical background to the debate, as well as offering practical insight into the questions which medical staff have to face when caring for patients who are seriously or incurably ill. They are thus partly based on scientific research and partly based on personal experiences and beliefs. They also enable valuable comparisons to be made between the situation in the UK and that in the Netherlands, where the argument is more advanced in terms of both public debate and the legislative structure.

The last chapter of the book is a record of the final plenary discussion of the symposium, and it addresses the central theme of whether there is a contradiction between palliative care and euthanasia, or whether eutha-nasia is simply a part, albeit a final one, of the range of care which medicine can offer to the sick.

There is no suggestion that nurses have a formal or an active part to play in the practice of euthanasia but, because the nurse usually has a closer relationship with the patient than any other member of the medical staff, her role in any discussion and decision-making may be crucial. This book may help nurses to form a personal perspective on the subject.

Contents

Hospice and Palliative Care 9
Elizabeth G Jones

Palliative Care: an Ethical Approach 17
Maureen McLellan

Euthanasia and the British Legislative Process 25
Janice Turner

The Law of Homicide in England and Wales 31
Susan A Hodge

Euthanasia: the Dutch Political Perspective 40
Leonard J van der Hout

Euthanasia and the Law in the Netherlands 49
Gusta van den Bogaard

Euthanasia: an Ethical Approach 55
Frank A Huser

Euthanasia as a Nursing Problem 63
Janny A Teule

Opposition, or towards a Continuum 68
Frank A Huser

The Authors 71

Hospice and Palliative Care

Elizabeth G Jones

The ideology of hospice begins with the vision that in the time before death there is often a surprising potential for personal and family growth, and that if a dying person is recognised as the unique individual he is, and enabled to live until he dies, with his maximum potential, he can still reach out to his hopes and expectations and to what has deepest meaning for him and end his life with a sense of completion. *(Saunders, 1993)*.

As the hospice movement in Britain receives increasing attention from European colleagues, this chapter aims to present brief details of the development of the hospice movement so positively promoted by Dame Cicely Saunders above; the meaning of palliative care; the services available, and possible future directions.

From Medieval times the word 'hospice' was used to describe a Christian institution where travellers and pilgrims could find food and shelter on their journey; it was not primarily associated with dying people. However, the sick and dying were also welcomed and cared for.

In Britain, a religious order, the Irish Sisters of Charity, began work in the late 19th and early 20th century in setting up homes for the incurably sick, the destitute and dying. St Joseph's Hospice in the east end of London was founded in 1905 and is where, in the 1950s, the founder of the 'modern hospice movement', Dame Cicely Saunders, worked as a doctor and began to develop techniques in pain control. Through research she established that better pain relief could be achieved by giving drugs such as diamorphine orally at regular intervals. Detailed control of symptoms, psychological care for patients and support for relatives were the key principles of care she observed *(Lewis, 1992)* and these underpinned the philosophy of care when she founded St Christopher's Hospice in 1967 as the first research and teaching hospice.

In Britain, the 1960s saw great developments in the treatment and care for people with cancer. There were advances in the use of radiotherapy and chemotherapy which aimed to cure the disease, or to control it and relieve symptoms. The word 'palliative' stems from the Latin 'pallium' – to cloak, or cover – and is used to describe treatment which relieves distressing symptoms in a disease which itself remains incurable.

The 'philosophy of palliative care' is often used interchangeably with 'the philosophy of hospice care' as a concept of total care, or holistic care for patients with advanced cancer. This reflects the simultaneous growth of the hospice movement and advances in cancer treatments. Palliative care and hospice care are phrases which are sometimes used euphemistically for terminal care and this has led to a continued debate about when, and for whom palliative care is appropriate.

A useful definition of palliative care has been suggested by the World Health Organisation:

> 'The active, total care of patients whose disease is not responsive to curative treatment, control of pain, of other symptoms, and of psychological, social, and spiritual problems, is paramount. The goal of palliative care is achievement of the best quality of life for patients and their families.' (WHO,1990).

The European Association for Palliative Care offers five key objects :

- to affirm life and regard death as a normal process
- to neither hasten, nor postpone death
- to provide relief from pain and other distressing symptoms
- to integrate psychological and spiritual aspects of care
- to offer a support system to help the family cope during the patients illness, and afterwards, in bereavement.

(European Association of Palliative Care Constitution Milan, 1988)

There has been a subtle shift in recent years, from what was initially referred to as terminal care to what is now known as palliative care, culminating in 1987 with the recognition by the Royal College of Physicians of palliative medicine as a sub-speciality of general medicine.

Saunders (1993) uses the term to refer to appropriate treatment. even before a patient can be rightly termed 'dying', that can make a radical difference to life and death. Doyle (1993) sought to clarify the practice of palliative medicine, by considering it to be the study and management of patients with active, progressive and advanced disease for whom the prognosis is limited. This would exclude patients with long term but stable chronic illness.

Palliative care as a multidisciplinary concept starts with the recognition that a cure will not be possible and that the emphasis of treatment should change from the pursuit of a cure to the provision of care.

If this is not acknowledged the result may be the continuation of vigorous and invasive treatment which, in the absence of improvement, causes anxiety and distress to the patient and family. However, the decision of when to discontinue such efforts will be different for each patient, as each poses a unique case. Patients with a terminal illness need appropriate therapy and treatment throughout the course of their illness. At one stage therapy is diverted towards investigation and intervention in order to control and/or cure such illness and alleviate associated symptoms. For some, the time comes when cure and remission are beyond the capacity of current curative treatment. In general, palliative care requires limited use of apparatus and technology, extensive personal care, and an ordering of the physical and social environment to be therapeutic in itself.

Kearney (1992) says that palliative care is not just symptomatology, when illness is seen as a problem to be solved. He says that suffering can have a meaning and a value, that there is potential in such an experience. What is important is the quality of the relationship between the professional and the patient that is of itself 'of healing value' (that is, healing in the sense of enabling a person to feel whole and at peace with himself).

But palliative care is not nursing and psychological care alone. Changes may occur throughout an illness which make a patient a candidate for active medical intervention once again. The everyday practice of palliative care raises complex moral issues. When should radical curative treatment be stopped? What steps should be taken when food and drink can no longer be taken by mouth? Ashby and Stoffell (1991) explain how different modes of care are appropriate at different stages of the disease process.

The 'curative mode' is the phase of therapeutic intervention in the course of a disease in which cure or complete remission is a realistic expectation. Prolongation of life and survival are the aims and a high rate of treatment related toxicity and morbidity may be acceptable. Comfort is a secondary issue; when a comfort measure conflicts with survival, the supremacy of survival is the dominant theme.

The 'palliative mode' is a phase in the course of a disease in which curative treatment is not expected to prolong life, and in which the benefits of treatment may be outweighed by its toxicity. Therapeutic interventions are directed at the supremacy of comfort, symptom relief, and general well-being.

The 'terminal mode' is the phase in which death seems inevitable and imminent. There is clinical evidence of the final part of the dying process, including poor appetite, weight loss, failure of physiological systems, and progression of the disease. The process of anticipatory grief may have commenced for both patient and family. The intake of food and fluid decreases, no form of artificial hydration or nutrition is undertaken and all measures not required for comfort are withdrawn.

A precise point of transition may not always occur and patients need the chance to discuss the pesonal benefits and costs of continuing with treatment. However carers and relatives often fear that if patients are confronted with the truth they will become depressed and give up the will to live. Saunders (1993) believes that there needs to be some degree of shared awareness of the true situation if a patient is to be enabled to live his remaining life to the full, rather than alone with his fears.

The transition between these modes of care is blurred (as has been described) and until recently palliative care has been limited to patients with a confirmed diagnosis of advanced cancer and whose life expectancy is short. It is arguable however, that palliative care is equally appropriate for patients with other diseases, such as AIDS; and also that the philosophy and principles can equally be transferred to settings other than hospice - they can be applied wherever dying patients are cared for. Patients with motor neurone disease have been cared for at several hospices since the early days, possibly because like malignant cancer it is an incurable, rapidly progressive disease with a predictable prognosis.

Harris (1990) talks of the 'disadvantaged dying', – those patients who have not been identified as having a terminal illness; or those in the terminal phase of a chronic illness, such as chronic obstructive airways disease, where the 'terminal phase' is difficult to define. These patients may not be referred for specialist services or admitted to a hospice. Harris argues that there has been a disproportionate concentration on those dying of cancer and this has created an underclass of dying people who have an equal claim to the resources and expertise to improve their quality of life. This is an issue of current debate and some hospices and palliative care teams are extending their services to include non-cancer patients.

However, the proportion of people with terminal cancer who receive any form of specialist hospice service is probably no more than 10% (*Clark, 1994*), and there has been a significant change in ideas about the models of care which hospices might best develop in order to make services more accessible. Indeed the philosophy of 'hospice' is founded not in the physical building of but in the application of principles of hospice-type care to a variety of settings whenever patients may be dying.

A research study by Townsend and Frank (1990) provides evidence that, given the choice, 58% of terminally ill cancer patients would prefer to die at home, but only 24% of those in the study actually did so; 20% wished to die in a hospital, but 56% did so; and 20% of those interviewed said they would choose to die in a hospice, but 7% did so.

Having a choice in where one dies is seen as an important aspect in maximising the quality of life experienced by dying patients, but as long ago as 1952 the Marie Curie Memorial Foundation published a report detailing a great deal of suffering among patients dying of cancer at home. The first hospice home-care team was established in 1969 to provide symptom control advice and emotional support, to compliment the care given by community staff. In recent years, with the financial support and education backing of the Cancer Relief Macmillan Fund the number of 'Macmillan Nurses' has grown to enable more patients to remain at home and die peacefully.

As Dunlop and Hockley (1991) discuss, even a hospice is not necessarily the best place for everyone and much distress may be caused to patients when they are pressurised into entering hospices (as is reported to happen as a way of making more hospital beds available for the acutely ill.) It is part of the philosophy of hospice care that the pursuit of research and education to promote new and positive attitudes should enable the skills of palliative care to be practised in a variety of settings, but the *ad hoc* way in which this has happened – due largely to public demand – was not foreseen in the early days of hospice care.

In 1993, throughout the whole of the United Kingdom there were 193 in-patient units, providing almost 2993 beds; 360 home care teams working from hospital, hospice and community bases; 186 day care hospices, either free-standing or attached to a hospice, and over 160 hospitals with terminal care support teams or support nurses (*St Christopher's Hospice Information Service (1993)*.

Following a review of palliative care services available in one Health Authority in 1991, the South West Thames Regional Health Authority proposed a model of comprehensive palliative care to include the following elements:

- in-patient hospice care
- in-patient hospital care
- hospital support team
- day services
- home care
- community care by primary health care teams
- bereavement counselling
- formal education
- informal education and advice
- other voluntary support.

(South West Regional Health Authority (1991)

Today, the majority of specialist services are provided through the voluntary sector and charities, although there are a number of hospices wholly operated by the National Health Service and the community services provided through the Macmillan Cancer Relief Fund (which is a charity) have strong links into the National Health Service infrastructure. As the development of voluntary hospice service has grown, so too has the call for statutory funding to be increased and significant change has taken place in the past five years with the commitment of central government to increase statutory finding in response to the case put forward by the hospice movement for financial help. By 1991 it was estimated that the cost of providing services approached £½ billion per annum. With these levels of provision and expenditure it became imperative for the many small independent and NHS units which comprise the hospice movement to present a united voice to the public and government. In 1991 the National Council for Hospice and Specialist Palliative Care Services, the 'National Hospice Council' was established with three main objectives: to represent the views and interests of hospice organisations and palliative care teams to government departments and to the media and public; to provide advice and assistance to hospice organisations and palliative care teams in their relations with health authorities; and to provide a general advisory service in all matters that require co-ordination or are of national interest and concern, such as taxation, legislation, charity issues, statutory funding, insurance and health and safety.

The National Council publishes occasional papers offering guidelines for good practice. In response to the implementation of the community care legislation in April 1993, it recommended standards for Health Authorities and Social Services departments for care in the community for people who are terminally ill. This legislation means that the elderly, the sick and dying, will be cared for in their own homes much more than at present, by the increase in provision of community nursing services and social services. As research has shown, patient's own preferences are for remaining at home to die. This suggests that in future their wishes are more likely to be met.

Conclusion

The hospice movement has been instrumental in dramatically improving the care of dying patients in the UK. The original aim of the movement was to create a new approach to the care of dying people, and it was created in response to the perception that the needs of dying patients and their families were not being met within the mainstream care provided by the National Health Service. There have been major changes in the way health and social care are provided by the state which will mean that hospices will need to review their own 'model' of care. Nowadays there is an increased emphasis on domiciliary and day care services, along with various 'outreach' programmes designed to make services more accessible.

This has coincided with greater interest in rehabilitation, and in support for family carers by respite provision as well as visual care such as sitting and befriending services.

There is a heightened emphasis on quality issues, cost effectiveness and equity, and hospices will be under more pressure to demonstrate their effectiveness. Independent hospices have had a high level of autonomy but if they are more closely linked to the National Health Service by service contracts as the legislation proposes, then there will be more regulation over future development. As Clark (1994) says 'it is now time to embrace the notion of a "second wave" of hospice development, through clarification of key strategic goals and a plan for their achievement'. Hospices are at the cross-roads.

References

Ashby M, Stoffell B., 1991 *Therapeutic ratio and defined phrases : proposal of ethical framework for palliative care* BMJ 302, 1322-1324

Clark   D, 1994 *At the cross-roads: which direction for the hospices?* Palliative Medicines 8, 1-3

Doyle D, 1993 *Palliative medicine – a time for definition* Palliative Medicine 7, 4, Editorial

Doyle D, Hanks G, MacDonald N, (editors) 1993. *Textbook of Palliative Medicine* New York, Oxford University Press

Dunlop R, Hockley J, 1991 *The distress of inappropriate Hospice Transfer* Palliative Medicine 5, 1, 61-61

European Association for Palliative Care, Vicolo Fiori 2, Milan Italy

Kearney M, 1992 *Palliative Care – just another speciality* Palliative Medicine 6, 1, 39-46

Lewis M, 1989 *Tears and smiles. The Hospice Handbook* London, Michael O'Mara Books Ltd.

Marie Curie Memorial Foundation 1952 *Report on a National Survey concerning patients nursed at house* London, Marie Curie Foundation.

Townsen, J, Frank A, et al 1990 *Terminal Cancer Care and Patient's preference for a place of death, a prospective study* BMJ September 301, 415-417

Saunders C, 1993 Foreword in Doyle D et al (editors) *The Oxford Textbook of Palliative Medicine* New York. Oxford University Press.

South West Thames Regional Authority 1992. *Palliative Care Contracts, Regional Guidelines* London South West Thames Regional Health Authority.

St Christopher's Hospice Information Service 1993. *Directory of Hospice Services* London. St Christopher's Hospice

World Health Organisation 1990. *Cancer Pain Relief and Palliative Care* Technical Report Series 804. Geneva.

Palliative Care: an Ethical Approach

Maureen McLellan

To everything there is a season,
and a time for every purpose
under heaven. — Ecclesiastes 3:1

It is not the intention of this chapter to explore in depth the theoretical tenets of principlism, or to enter the dialogue which currently seeks to examine the appropriateness or applicability of ethical principlism in the arena of health care. Nor is it proposed to present, in detail, an alternative ethical perspective which is under consideration, particularly in relation to health care, and which centres on an analysis of the concept of caring and the ethical issues which emanate from activities associated with caring.

The paper will present an overview of these stances, and will offer a palliative care perspective on the ethical issues which commonly arise for practitioners. It is the contention here that the philosophy which under-pins palliative care practice successfully incorporates ethical principlism within ethical caring in order to address and reduce suffering, and in doing presents an acceptable alternative to those who believe that euthanasia is the answer to unnecessary suffering.

Interest in biomedical ethics has grown significantly over recent years. This seems to have arisen out of the fact that medical technology is developing rapidly. The 'medicalisation' of life and living has reached such a stage that health care practitioners are required to address an ever increasing number of ethical dilemmas posed by the everyday practice of medicine and nursing. These dilemmas range from issues of confidentiality and informed consent, through to the major ethical dilemmas associated with the beginning and ending of life itself. Ethicists believe that the application of ethical thinking to such complex situations will facilitate the establishment of behavioural norms and therefore guide practitioners in their decision making.

Currently the predominant approach to medical ethics links with 'principlism'. This approach involves a set of rules and principles which have been derived from various schools of ethical thinking. The bases of principlism are thought to be valid for all human beings, of all ages, throughout the world.

The object of applying ethical principles to medical and/or nursing situations is to enable practitioners to separate out relevant issues and come to a decision which will be morally acceptable. The problem with morals, of course, is that they exist! Moral codes vary according to personal, societal and cultural norms and may not be universally acceptable. In view of this, the application of these universal principles to complex ethical dilemmas should facilitate decision making and guide behaviour in situations, which by their very nature, are inherently difficult to deal with.

The major principles involved in this approach include the principle of non-maleficence and the principle of justice.

It should be borne in mind that these principles are not considered to be absolute, but are *prima facie* binding. To illustrate this point Beauchamp and Childress outline the thesis presented by W.D. Ross which posits a pluralistic deontological approach in situations involving conflict and judgement. Ross believed that where there is a conflict of principles the over-riding duty is uncovered by locating the greatest balance of right over wrong. Thus which principle overrides in a case of conflict will depend on the context under consideration.

It is also important to note that if it is acceptable that these principles form the basis of what have been called 'laws of humanity', then they apply equally to all human beings. Thus, my right to self determination through autonomous choice is only acceptable as long as it does not compromise the autonomy of another human being.

Critics of this approach propose that the application of such abstract, and often conflicting, principles to the human situation only serves to minimalise the dilemmas facing the individuals who are grappling with the reality of a given situation. They suggest that, rather than adhere to rigid principles, we return to the common bond that unites us all – our humanity. The argument proposed is that if we learn to accept and act on this common bond, then we will care for and about others simply because we share with them our basic humanity. This view is currently receiving significant consideration. In particular, one American anthropologist has developed the work of Gilligan and contends that 'caring means considering the other, his/her nature and way of life, his/her needs and desires and trying to apprehend the reality of his/her existence.'

Noddings argues that the commitment to act on behalf of the cared for, a continued interest in his/her reality throughout the appropriate time span, and the continued renewal of commitment over this span of time, are essential elements of caring.

For health care professionals the caring relationship should be characterised by 'receptivity' where within a trusting relationship, there is acceptance and positive regard for the cared for, 'relatedness' where the individual is recognised as an expert on his/her own reality and practitioners recognise that 'patients' are their raison d'être and 'responsiveness' where practitioners should be responsive to need, in presence with the individual, and focused on the time and situation.

Having reviewed both of these ethical approaches it is probably apparent to the reader that there may be limitations in each, and that perhaps the wisest course of action would be to combine the approaches to produce an ethical framework which simultaneously provides structure, sensitivity and flexibility.

The original contention of this paper was that palliative care incorporates philosophical tenets from both of the ethical approaches previously described. To examine this contention it is necessary to consider the nature and function of palliative care practice.

Palliative care is not concerned with mechanistic views of the body. Roy illustrates this point poignantly in the following lines –

> 'Palliative and hospice care, conceived in the crucible of dying cancer patient neglect, is one of the modern period's most powerful challenges to unwitting splits of the mind from the body; of cure from care; of patient from family; of family from society; and of scientific objectivity from human compassion. The governing idea of palliative and hospice care has been "see, not just disease, not just the patient, but the person in his and her totality and total particularity".'

Thus, in situations where physical disintegration is often the norm, there exists a philosophy of care which determines that any individual will be considered in his or her entirety – as an integrated human being who in his dying has the potential to attain and maintain the ultimate integrity which results from having completed the process of living.

Defining the boundaries of palliative care has proved extraordinarily difficult over the years. This difficulty stems from the fact that we will die one day. Dying is part of living and, therefore, should not become an unnecessarily abnormal process. The following definition offered by the World Health Organisation demonstrates the nature and extent of palliative care.

Palliative care is the active care of patients whose disease is not responsive to curative treatment. Control of pain, of other symptoms, and of psychological, social and spiritual problems is paramount. The goal of palliative care is achievement of the best possible quality of life for patients and their families. Many aspects of palliative care are also applicable earlier in the course of the illness, in conjunction with anti cancer treatment. Palliative care:

- affirms life and regards dying as a normal process;
- neither hastens nor postpones death;
- provides relief from pain and other distressing symptoms;
- integrates the psychological and spiritual aspects of patient care;
- offers a support system to help patients live as actively as possible until death;
- offers a support system to help the family cope during the patient's illness and in their own bereavement.

Obviously great sensitivity is required by health care professionals who are caring for people at the point where they are informed that curative treatment has no further part to play in the fight against their condition. From this point, the relationship between practitioner and the individual and his/her family is activated. It is vital that throughout the time span between prognosis and death this relationship, which is founded on mutual trust and must be developed through continuing mutual respect and honesty, is one which constitutes a partnership between professionals and the dying person and his family as the unit of care.

This open and honest relationship forms an ethical basis for the delivery and receipt of palliative care. The unconditional acceptance and affirmation of the patient's value as a person reminds practitioners of the need to help individuals to maintain dignity and personal integrity, in spite of apparent disintegration and the resulting potential for loss of dignity.

The cornerstones of successful palliative care involve symptom control, psycho social care, teamwork and partnership between patient/family and professionals. The goal of palliative care is comfort as defined by the dying person.

Despite this fundamentally ethical approach to care which incorporates the principles of autonomy, beneficence, and veracity encompassed in a philosophy of care which addresses receptivity, relatedness and responsitivity, ethical dilemmas arise and require attention. As with mainstream health care the issues are many and various.

However, for the purpose of this paper, these are summarised in Table 1 and only some of the more major issues will be discussed.

Wilkinson also notes that there are special features relating to ethical issues in palliative care. These include the fact that the patient may be frail, weak and possibly confused. This will render him/her vulnerable and in need of special care. By virtue of diagnosis and prognosis, the

Table 1 - Summary of ethical issues in palliative care

I *Issues of care and comfort*	1 Professional - patient relationship 2 Transition to palliative care 3 Control of symptoms 4 Principle of double effect
II *Issues of consent and communication*	1 Consent 2 Research 3 Confidentiality 4 Disclosure
III *Issues of life and death*	1 Prolongation of life 2 Termination of life
IV *Issues of needs and resources*	1 Cost of health care 2 Provision of health care 3 Allocation of resources
V *Issues of HIV infection*	

Source: Wilkinson, J. 1993

dying person may be subject to fears and anxieties which may affect behaviour and thus call for a sensitive approach to spiritual care. Relatives must also be considered and given their due place in the management of care and the ability to cope with practical matters before and after death. Some of the major ethical issues which may arise will now be discussed.

Symptom control

The prevention and control of distressing symptoms is one of the principal functions of palliative medicine.

Control of suffering in patients experiencing the overwhelming distress of some physical symptoms is not always easy, and at times requires intensive and extraordinary pharmacological intervention. Care is structured around responding to need as defined by the patient with the principle of beneficence guiding action. Practitioners involved in hospice or palliative care can all recall instances where, once physical suffering is controlled requests for euthanasia or the desire for suicide are no longer discussed. Instead, the dying person is able to achieve a level of personal integrity and acceptance which appears to result from the knowledge that he or she will be cared for in dying.

Prolongation of life

The goal of palliative care is patient comfort. Extraordinary measures which seek to prolong the distress of dying are not appropriate. Prolongation of life at all costs is also inappropriate. The medical power to do good has reached its limits when prolonging dying is all it can achieve. Thus, allowing the dying to die, and taking all care to ensure that they do not die in pain and distress, but in a peaceful and dignified manner also utilise the principle of beneficence within the context of caring.

Termination of life

The debate surrounding this issue is a central consideration of this symposium, and there are no easy answers. Those who seek to advance the practice of euthanasia do so on the basis of humanity and unnecessary suffering. Is the answer to unnecessary suffering the elimination of the sufferer or the elimination of the cause of the suffering? The principle of autonomy is not absolute. Such a request from a patient, which implies that the doctor acts against his or her will, compromises the doctor's right to make an autonomous choice. Furthermore, legalisation of euthanasia would eventually compromise the autonomy of the community at large. How many disabled, elderly or infirm members of society may be insidiously pressured into feeling that they were too great a burden on society? How many may be persuaded that they should seek euthanasia for the societal good? How does this equate with pre-war and war time practices in Nazi Germany? And how many voices have been raised in horror that such atrocities were allowed to occur then?

On the basis of our common humanity, we cannot condone such a practice. It goes far beyond medical and societal mandates and when examining the issue according to pluralistic deontology, it is difficult to locate the balance of right over wrong.

Justice in the use of resources
Given the current economic climate and the fact that health care needs are infinite while resources are finite, it is necessary to consider needs in relation to resources using an appropriate ethical decision making framework. In the UK this is difficult enough, even when resources are relatively plentiful. However, the global situation may be vastly different, particularly when resources are scarce. Nevertheless, the appropriate distribution of resources, whether scarce or plentiful, is dependent upon three factors; the personal integrity of those involved in resource allocation, the accurate identification of need and the consideration of needs and resources in the light of an agreed ethical framework. This is never easy and seldom seen to be right and just by all parties concerned. However, as health care workers we are stewards of available resources, and are to a greater or lesser extent responsible for determining their effective use and justifiable ethical allocation.

In conclusion, I have argued that the philosophy of palliative care incorporates the best of principlism and the caring ethic. Despite the fact that this paper has only dealt at a superficial level with issues which in their own right are worthy of considerable debate, the emerging impression is of a situation where two apparently diverse ethical stances live in peaceful co-existence. The resulting ethical framework enables practitioners to provide a level of care which is concerned with the reduction of suffering and quality of life.

To suggest that this level of care and attention to the reduction of suffering is universally available would be erroneous. Each of us knows of at least one situation where suffering is not relieved. This is unacceptable. Palliative care practitioners have a professional responsibility to rectify this situation through educational and research endeavours. However, there is a concomitant responsibility which requires that all health care practitioners are open to the suggested changes in practice which result from such endeavours.

To those who argue that suffering is unnecessary in life I would say that we should remember that suffering like death is part of life. The abrupt end to suffering, brought about through the abrupt ending of life sacrifices the life in the cause of the suffering.

Surely it would be more logical to develop ways of preventing some of the suffering and relieving the remainder, in order that human beings are freed from the suffering which dominates consciousness and prevents them from becoming all that they can be and taking hold of the opportunities life affords.

While I do not disagree that clinical medicine is in a period of 'paradigmatic instability', I would argue that palliative medicine has achieved a paradigmatic shift and adopts a philosophy which constantly seeks to provide comfort and relieve suffering. Thus, it is my final contention that the answer to the unnecessary suffering referred to by the pro-euthanasia lobby appears to lie in the development of palliative care services and not in the legalisation of euthanasia.

I started this chapter with some words from Ecclesiastes which urges us to remember that there is a 'time for every purpose under heaven.'

Given the context of this symposium, I now leave you with the following words which may provide some food for thought.

> *Men are disturbed, not by things that happen, but by their opinion of the things that happen.* — Epictetus

Euthanasia and the British Legislative Process

Janice Turner

This chapter explains the parliamentary procedures available in Britain to individual MPs who wish to attempt to change the law on euthanasia and outlines the various attempts that have been made over the last 60 years. It discusses some of the problems faced by such MPs and why legislation on such sensitive issues is left to back bench MPs to introduce.

Following the publication of the Report of the House of Lords Select Committee on Medical Ethics (1994), it is extremely unlikely that in the foreseeable future there will be any government bill to change the law on euthanasia despite the pleas of the Law Lords after the Bland case. However, even before this Report, it was always highly unlikely that any attempt to change the law would be a party political issue espoused by the government of the day.

There is a long tradition in the British legislative process of certain types of legislation, especially those which deal with matters of individual morality or conscience, being introduced by individual Members of Parliament as opposed to the government itself – for example, the legalisation of homosexuality, the abolition of capital punishment, abortion reform and the liberalisation of the divorce laws all resulted from private members' legislation. As McDonald (1989) states:

'Governments normally prefer to leave it to private member's legislation to deal with highly controversial moral issues or social reforms on matters of individual morality, mainly because members of their own party, both inside or outside parliament, hold conflicting views on such issues and tend to regard them as a question of individual conscience rather than party ideology'.

Thus, in order to understand past attempts to change the law on euthanasia and to predict the possibility of success in the future, it is necessary to understand the procedures open to MPs as Private Members to introduce legislation. By convention, 'Private Members' are backbenchers in both the House of Commons and House of Lords. Ministers and Opposition front-bench spokesmen and women are thus excluded from the definition.

Hanson and Walles (1990) point out that 'The House of Commons is essentially a body in which the back bench Members ratify decisions taken elsewhere', and for the majority of the business which is put before the House, this is undoubtedly true. During the 160 days on which the House sits and which generally comprise a Parliamentary session, about 90% of the time is spent on government business (which includes both government and official opposition) leaving 10% for Private Members business *(Madgwick, 1984)*.

About half of the time that the House sits is devoted to the process of the various stages necessary to the enactment of legislation (excluding committee time where bills are examined in detail) and most of that time is given over to government legislation *(Hanson and Walles, 1990)*. Government Bills are, of course, usually successful, exceptions to the general rule of government supremacy – such as the defeat of the 1986 Shops Bill following the defection of 72 Conservative backbenchers – being very rare *(Hanson and Walles, 1990)*. Thus, 'From his mid-nineteenth century ascendancy, the Private member has been relegated in terms of legislative initiative to a very minor place" *(ibid)*.

In this 'minor place' Private Members are able, under certain procedures, to introduce Private Members Bills (PMBs) in a variety of ways. Firstly, they can use the twelve Fridays which are made available in each parliamentary session. Given the demand from MPs so to do, and the limited time available, selection of which Bills are brought forward depends upon success in the ballot held at the beginning of the session. Over 400 MPs are eligible to enter the ballot from which twenty names are drawn. However, only the first six or so drawn are assured of the opportunity for a debate on their bills.

There are many hurdles that a PMB has to overcome on its way to the statute book. These include drafting the bill, getting through all the necessary procedural stages and surviving the variety of devices that opponents may use to obstruct and destroy the Bill (devices such as 'talking the bill out' by keeping the debate going past four o'clock without the question being put, tabling a large number of amendments, or delaying the bill at the committee stage to prevent it being able to complete all its stages within the parliamentary session).

As McDonald (1989) says: 'On an issue which is a matter of deeply held conviction for all concerned, both sides will use every Parliamentary procedure open to them to achieve their aims'.

What all this means in essence is that for a PMB to be successful it has to be non-controversial and/or have at least tacit Government support *(Adonis, 1993)*. The Government may give support because it believes that there is strong feeling both inside and outside the House or because they support the principle of the bill *(McDonald, 1989)*. It may then facilitate the bill's passage by ensuring it has adequate parliamentary time, as happened for example, with PMBs on the abolition of capital punishment and abortion reform. Marsh and Reed's (1988) study of PMBs showed that only when this happens can PMBs ever be successful.

An MP may also be allowed to propose a bill under the 'ten minute rule' when he or she is given the opportunity to make a ten minute speech proposing the introduction of a bill. The times set aside for this are Tuesdays and Wednesdays, from the seventh week of the session, immediately after Question Time, when one bill each day may be proposed. Question Time occupies the first forty to fifty minutes of every sitting, Monday to Thursday.

During this period, specified Ministers appear, on a rota, before the House, to answer questions orally on their department's duties and activities. On Tuesdays and Thursdays, the Prime Minister has to answer questions for the last fifteen minutes of the Question Time period. The value of speaking under the ten minute rule is that, because it follows Question Time, the House and the press gallery are usually packed to capacity and the MP has access to prime media time (this is especially true of Prime Minister's Question Time on a Tuesday)*(Adonis, 1993)* although the House may sometimes empty quite quickly after question time.

In order to be able to propose a bill under this procedure, the MP has to queue to give notice of the bill at the Public Bills Office at 10 o'clock in the morning, usually three weeks in advance. He or she may well have to stay up all night in order to be first in the queue and thus be assured of the opportunity *(McDonald, 1989)*. After the MP has spoken, an opponent gives a ten minute speech in opposition, after which a vote is taken. If the vote is in favour of the bill, the proposer then introduces it to the House. Only twenty five ten minute rule bills have become law since 1945 and none since 1983/4 *(Garrett, 1992)*.

A third way in which a PMB may be introduced is under the procedure known as 'Ordinary Presentation under Standing Order 58'. In this case, a bill is introduced but not debated and therefore there is generally little or no publicity. In order to use this procedure, the MP simply has to give notice the previous day. Bills may be introduced on any sitting day after the fifth Wednesday of the session. One successful example of legislation resulting from this procedure was the 1985 Act prohibiting female circumcision.

Backbenchers in the House of Lords can also introduce PMBs – more easily, in fact, than their Commons counterparts. However, as with other PMBs, such bills will only succeed if having been passed by the Lords they are either uncontroversial or have government support.

Marsh and Reed's research (cited in Adonis, 1993) revealed that, during the 1983–87 Parliament, the overall success rate of PMBs was 15%. Individual success rates under the various procedures outlined above were as follows:

> 49% of balloted bills – 39 successful bills
> 1% of ten minute rule bills – 2 successful bills
> 12% of Standing Order 58 bills – 13 successful bills
> 23% of private peers bills – 14 successful bills

Despite the difficulty of PMBs becoming law without being either uncontroversial or having government support, Adonis (1993) argues that PMBs

> 'provide an important mechanism enabling the major parties, between them, to agree on legislation affecting delicate social and moral issues while respecting the conscience of backbenchers and keeping their leaders free of binding commitments' and that as such 'their utility should not be underestimated' (p110).

However, the value of PMBs is not simply to be measured in terms of their success or otherwise in reaching the statute book. Simply by introducing a PMB, an MP is given the opportunity to raise an issue that she or he feels strongly about, to test opinion in the House and the publicity that may arise may be valuable in the longer term in changing opinion by contributing to a wider debate and discussion of the issues, even if, in the short term, no legislative change occurs. Unsuccessful PMBs have often paved the way for future change – for example, the private peer's bill which failed in 1989 to restrict the hours worked by junior hospital doctors, raised public awareness of the issue and led to eventual, if limited change by the government *(Adonis,1993)*.

Thus, it might be argued that unsuccessful parliamentary attempts to legalise euthanasia in certain circumstances and with certain safeguards, over the last sixty years, have contributed to the general debate of the issues involved and have helped to raise overall awareness.

However, such attempts to change the law also mirror a body of opinion outside parliament and it was no coincidence that the first bill to be introduced that dealt with euthanasia, the Voluntary Euthanasia (Legalisation) Bill, introduced in 1936 as a PMB in the House of Lords by Lord Ponsonby, had speedily followed the founding in 1935 of the Voluntary Euthanasia Legalisation Society (VELS). The VELS was established by a group of churchmen, lawyers and eminent doctors including Lord Moynihan, its first President, who was also President of the Royal College of Surgeons.

The 1936 bill was rejected at the second reading, which is the stage during which the principles of a bill are debated. A contribution to that debate was made by Lord Dawson of Penn, one of the royal doctors, who argued that legalisation was not necessary since good doctors already helped their patients to die if the occasion arose. It later transpired that he was speaking from personal experience, having ended the life of King George V earlier that year with pain-killing injections *(VES, 1993)*.

Since 1936, there have been similar unsuccessful attempts to introduce PMBs in the House of Lords. Lord Chorley's motion to raise the issue of voluntary euthanasia in 1950 had a long debate but no vote, whilst in 1969 Lord Raglan's PMB on voluntary euthanasia was rejected. In 1985, the same fate befell Lord Jenkin's Suicide Act (1961) Amendment Bill which aimed to remove compassionate assistance to suicide as a crime.

As part of the wider issue, there have also been attempts, again in the Lords, to address the status of advance directives. In 1976 Baroness Wootton tried unsuccessfully, with her Incurable Patients Bill, to provide for advance directives refusing treatment and allowing adequate pain relief despite the consequences. Lord Allen's Medical Treatment (Advance Directives) Bill in 1993 sought to confirm the legal status of advance directives. Consideration of the latter bill was the first activity of the All-Party Parliamentary Voluntary Euthanasia Group set up in 1991 with members from both Houses and all major political parties.

It is interesting to note that it was not until 1990 that an attempt was made under the ten minute rule procedure to introduce a PMB dealing with euthanasia in the House of Commons. This motion, introduced by Roland Boyes MP, to bring in a bill to permit voluntary euthanasia was defeated by 101 votes to 35. A similar attempt in 1993 by Piara Khabra met a similar fate. Yet according to Helme (1991) there appears to be considerable support for the principle of active voluntary euthanasia as evidenced both by surveys of public attitudes (suggesting three-quarters of those questioned are in favour) and supportive academic and professional opinion. However, the House of Lords Report and the government's response to it appear to rule out the possibility of any successful attempts in the near future to change the law on euthanasia. The government appears to strongly support the Lords' Select Committee in their rejection of the case for legalising euthanasia but does draw a fine line between mercy killing and treatment decisions by doctors that result in death as a side-effect *(The Observer, 8 May 1994)*.

The debate, in many ways, appears to be back at square one – from where, no doubt, a private member will once again attempt to bring it forward.

References

Adonis A, 1993, *Parliament Today* Manchester University Press, Manchester.

Garrett J 1992, *Westminster. Does Parliament Work?* Gollanz, London

Hanson A H and Walles M, 1990, *Governing Britain (5th edition)* Fontana, London.

Helme T, 1991, *The Voluntary Euthanasia (Legalisation) Bill (1936) revisited.* Journal of Medical Ethics 17, 25-29

Madgwick PJ, 1984, *Introduction to British Politics (3rd edition)* Stanley Thornes, Cheltenham

McDonald O, 1989, *Parliament at Work* Methuen, London

Voluntary Euthanasia Society, 1993, *A Brief History Of the Voluntary Euthanasia Society* VES, London

The Law of Homicide in England and Wales

Susan A Hodge

Summary

The paper provides a brief summary of the nature of the law. The law relating to homicide is explained in its various forms and applied to the problems of treatment or non-treatment encountered by health-care professionals. Recent case law is analysed, highlighting the difficulties encountered by the courts in applying legal principles to ethical problems.

The law in England

English law today comes from two main sources. One source is case-law or precedent – that is, the decisions of the courts over the past centuries whereby legal principles have been explained in the light of the facts of particular cases. Precedent has allowed the evolution of what is known as the common law since 1066. Only Parliament can change the common law by means of legislation; the courts cannot do so although there is gradual development as new sets of circumstances arise which have not previously been considered by the judges.

The second main source is legislation (also referred to as statute law or Acts of Parliament) which is law created by the exercise of the democratic will as evidenced in Parliament. Parliament is sovereign and legislation cannot be challenged or questioned in the courts. The courts do have a role in interpreting what legislation actually means, but this is confined to finding the intention of Parliament as evidenced only by the words used in the statute.

Development of the common law and interpretation of statutes can only be undertaken by the courts once an action is brought to the courts by an aggrieved individual. There is generally no mechanism whereby the opinion of the court can be obtained simply because difficulty is anticipated.

Under English law the concept of euthanasia does not as such exist. Anyone who carries out such an act may well be charged with a serious criminal offence such as murder (a common law offence) or manslaughter. Thus those who are concerned with the care of the dying patient or who care for those suffering a painful and/or incurable illness must be aware of where the line between good practice within the law and criminal conduct will be drawn.

Murder

Murder is committed by any person who unlawfully kills a human being with malice aforethought, the death occurring within a year and a day of the act which causes it.

Under English law, the concept of 'malice aforethought' can be defined as an intention on the part of the accused person to kill the victim. A conviction for murder carries a mandatory sentence of life imprisonment.

Manslaughter

Involuntary manslaughter is committed where the accused has killed someone, but in circumstances where the law recognises that the accused's power of reasoning was so seriously impaired, for example by provocation or diminished responsibility, that the accused ought to be excused[1]. Involuntary manslaughter occurs where an act or omission by the accused results in the death of the victim. The accused does not intend to kill or cause serious bodily harm but does an act or omits to act with gross negligence or recklessly as to the possibility that death or serious injury may result.

Manslaughter is punished at the discretion of the judge with a maximum possible sentence of life imprisonment.

Intention

The fundamental difference between the crimes of murder and manslaughter stems from the mental attitude of the accused at the time of the killing. This is a matter for the jury to decide, having regard to all the evidence including what the accused says was the intended result or purpose. The fact that another person would have known or realised that death or serious injury was a likely result of the action by the accused does not mean that the accused also knew or intended this although it is clearly a factor of some weight where the risk is high. The jury must be satisfied that the accused intended to kill or cause really serious injury; this alone will suffice for a conviction of murder.[2]

In recent cases involving a health-care professional, juries have been prepared to give the professional the benefit of any doubt which exists, but nonetheless in a clear case the jury will convict.

In R v Arthur[3] a paediatrician was charged with the attempted murder of a Down's Syndrome infant whom he believed (as was later confirmed) also to be suffering from untreatable cardiac and other abnormalities. The accused prescribed dihydrocodeine and nursing care only, which would have led to the infant's death from starvation. He was however acquitted of the charge. In R v Cox[4] a consultant was charged with attempted murder after the death of a woman in the terminal stages of illness and allegedly suffering intense pain to whom he had given potassium chloride. Dr Cox was convicted of the offence charged.

Provocation and diminished responsibility
In reality neither of these defences are likely to be pleaded by health-care professionals whose patients have died. Provocation may be a defence where the accused suffered a sudden and temporary loss of self-control as a result of which and during which the murder occurred in circumstances where a reasonable person would, in the opinion of the jury, have acted similarly.

Diminished responsibility is often raised as a defence by relatives and other informal carers who have caused the death of a loved one 'to end his or her suffering.' For the defence to succeed the accused must show that at the time 'he was suffering from such abnormality of mind.... as substantially impaired his mental responsibility for his acts and omissions'.[5]

Lord Parker CVJ explained this as a state of mind which severely affected the accused's ability to distinguish between and recognise right from wrong thus affecting the accused's will-power to control physical acts.[6] In a number of cases, reported only as news items in media, juries have found themselves able to acquit the accused of murder and convict of manslaughter where the accused has been suffering from stress or depression resulting from caring for the victim of seriously disabling or terminal disease.

Consequences for treatment decision
Assuming the health-care professional to be competent in the exercise of

professional skills and to lack homicidal intent, decisions frequently need to be made as to whether or not treatment should be undertaken or prolonged. If the decision is not properly reached, liability for homicide may result. In the absence of legislation on this issue, guidance as to what may be lawful can only be obtained from past cases which have reached the higher courts on appeal.

It must always be remembered that under English law, no matter what the motive, no matter that the patient consents, there is no defence for any person who does an act or who omits to act for the purpose of hastening the death of a patient.[7] However some acts will be lawful even if as a result death is hastened. Lord Donaldson MR has stated 'the use of drugs to reduce pain will often be fully justified, notwithstanding that this will hasten the moment of death. What can never be justified is the use of drugs or surgical procedures with the primary purpose of doing so.'[8]

The courts thus recognise that steps may be taken 'to relieve pain and suffering even if the measures....may incidentally shorten life.'[9]

Competent adults

The long-standing rule is that no treatment of any kind may be given to a person without a valid consent to that treatment. If no such consent has been given by a competent person, any treatment which is given will give rise to civil and criminal liability on the part of the health-care professional who carries it out.

Thus 'every adult has the right and capacity to decide whether or not he will accept medical treatment, even if a refusal may... lead to premature death. Furthermore, it matters not whether the reasons for the refusal were rational or irrational, unknown or even non-existent. This is so notwithstanding the very strong public interest in preserving the life and health of all citizens.'[10]

Where consent is refused there is little difficulty if the patient remains conscious as the matter can be further discussed. Difficulties arise where the patient subsequently becomes incapable, when the health-care professional may need to consider whether the refusal was intended to be maintained in the changed situation.

If the refusal was not intended to be maintained yet no treatment is given and the patient dies, there may be liability for manslaughter; if however the refusal was intended to be maintained, any treatment given may give rise to both civil and criminal liability for assault and battery. Relevant matters for consideration by the health-care professional include the extent to which the patient was subject to fatigue, shock or pain or to the influence of others which may have overborne the patient's will.[11]

Incompetent adults

Where a decision about treatment needs to be made in respect of an adult who lacks mental capacity, who is unconscious or who is otherwise incapable of making an autonomous decision, treatment may lawfully be given provided that as a matter of clinical judgement it is in the best interests of the patient. The responsibility for the decision remains with the practitioner who may consult the next of kin for information as to the likely wishes of the patient and as to the patient's personal circumstances.

The next of kin do not however have the right to consent or to refuse consent on the patient's behalf.[12]

The dying and the 'living dead'

The courts have not had difficulty in accepting that it is lawful for a decision to be taken to cease ventilation of a patient who is 'brain-stem dead', the law regarding such a person as dead. Similarly it is lawful to omit treatment where the patient's best interests are served by such omission.[13] Recently however, in what has become known as 'the Bland case'[14], the issue has arisen for the first time in the English courts as to whether or not artificial nutrition and hydration can be withdrawn from a patient who is in the condition known as persistent vegetation state (PVS).

The patient concerned, Anthony Bland, had been in such a state for over 3 years and medical opinion was unanimous that he might live for many years. The medical and nursing staff concerned with his care and his family were all certain that his best interest would be served by ceasing nutrition and hydration and thus allowing him to die. There was concern that this would amount to homicide and thus render the persons responsible for his care liable to prosecution under the criminal law.

The courts were asked to declare that the proposed course would not give rise to civil liability. If such declaration were granted, the likelihood of criminal liability being found would be almost non-existent. The matter eventually came before the Judicial Committee of the House of Lords where the issues of treatment of an incompetent adult were fully reviewed with reference to a patient in PVS.[15]

The judges endeavoured to avoid setting out general principles which could be of application in other cases although it is already apparent that in this they have not been totally successful.

It was accepted by all the judges that in England 'there is no absolute rule that the patient's life must be prolonged by...treatment or care, if available, regardless of the circumstances.'[16]

The question at issue was in essence, if it is lawful in the patient's best interests to refrain from futile treatment and yet it is unlawful to take active steps to cause death,[17] how could it be lawful to withdraw artificial nutrition and hydration with the intention of causing the death of the patient by starvation?

It is accepted that a positive act which is intended to end life is unlawful but that an omission to act is lawful when the act would be futile.[18] Lord Justice Goff argued that a doctor 'in discontinuing life support, is simply allowing his patient to die of his pre-existing condition.'[19] The decision that has to be made therefore is not 'whether it is in the best interests of the patient that he should die. The question is whether it is in the best interests of the patient that his life should be prolonged by the continuance of this form of medical treatment or care.'[20]

The judges were unanimous in their opinion that, in this particular case, the answer to that question was no. Accordingly it was declared that no civil liability would be incurred by the cessation of artificial nutrition and hydration as its continuance could not be said to be of benefit to or in the best interests of the patient.

The ethical issues
It is not the writer's purpose to consider ethical issues in depth; that is a matter for philosophers and society. However, the principles of ethics cannot be ignored (although it was clearly felt by the judges that they were not the appropriate authority to declare what those principles were and how they should be applied to such issues). Lord Justice Browne-Wilkinson stated that he had 'no doubt that it is for Parliament, not the courts, to decide the broader issues.'[21]

In the meantime the judges acknowledge that on these issues public opinion is divided, as is medical opinion. 'The moral, social and legal issues raised by this case should be considered by Parliament. The judges' function in this area of the law should be to apply the principles which society, through the democratic process, adopts, not to impose their standards on society. If Parliament fails to act, then judge-made law will of necessity through a gradual and uncertain process provide a legal answer to each new question as it arises. But in my judgment that is not the best way to proceed.'[22]

The future

The judges in Bland were at pains to try to limit their decision to the particular circumstances of Anthony Bland.

This approach has however already been shown to be less than totally successful. A case came before the Court of Appeal on 14th January 1994 concerning a PVS patient about whom medical opinion was not in all respects unanimous and in respect of whom the court was asked to declare that doctors caring for him would not be acting unlawfully if they omitted to re-insert a stomach tube which had come out. Although there had not been a full and impartial inquiry by the Official Solicitor representing the interests of the patient (as envisaged in Bland), the court granted the declaration requested.

In the course of that judgment, full details of which are not at the time of writing available, Sir Thomas Bingham MR stated that circumstances could be envisaged when there would be no time for any application to the court to be made and that full enquiry by the Official Solicitor was not a pre-requisite to a decision to withdraw artificial nutrition and hydration.[23] It appears that the development of judge-made law on this issue anticipated by Lord Justice Browne-Wilkinson in Bland has begun.

The necessity for judge-made law has become more likely, at least in the foreseeable future, by virtue of the fact that the all-party Select Committee of the House of Lords reporting on 16th February 1994 concluded that euthanasia must remain illegal and rejected the creation of a new offence of mercy-killing.[24]

Suicide

If it is unlawful to kill a patient even at the patient's own well-considered request, could the problem be solved by giving advice as to effective methods of suicide and perhaps a prescription for an appropriate quantity of a suitable drug? Although suicide has not been a criminal offence in England since the Suicide Act 1961, it remains a criminal offence to 'aid abet counsel or procure' another person to commit suicide.

While the rationale behind such an offence is clear, it does mean that a health-care professional who gives advice, for example as to the quantity of a drug needed to kill oneself, may be successfully prosecuted under the provisions of the Act.

Conclusion

While the competent adult can, by exercise of the right to refuse treatment, ensure that his/her own wishes are honoured, decisions relating to the incompetent person have inevitably to be taken by others. At the present time it can be argued that the law is uncertain, reflecting society's own uncertainties on these issues.

For the moment all that an individual can do to ensure that life is not maintained in circumstances unacceptable to that individual, is to make a 'living will' or an 'advanced directive.' This document, which has no legal force of itself, provides valuable evidence as to a patient's own wishes in the event that he or she becomes incapable of expressing an autonomous decision.

The legal duties of the health-care professionals involved do not change nor is the document conclusive of what constitutes the best interest of the patient. It has however been acknowledged by the courts that a living will constitutes valuable evidence to assist the health-care professional in reaching the extremely difficult decision to treat or not to treat or to withdraw treatment from a particular patient.[25]

References

1   *Homicide Act* 1957
2   *R v Moloney* (1985) 2 WLR 648
3   Reported in *The Times* 6th Nov 1981, cited in Kennedy & Grubb *Medical Law Text and Materials*
4   18th September 1992 unreported
5   *Homicide Act* 1957 s2
6   *R v Byrne* (1960) 2QB 396
7   Skegg *Law Ethics and Medicine*
8   In re J (a Minor) *Wardship: Medical Treatment* (1991) Fam. 33 p46
9   per Devlin J in *R v Bodkins-Adams* (1957) CLR 365
10 per Donaldson MR in re T *Adult: Refusal of Treatment* (1992) 3 WLR 799
11 In re T *Adult: Refusal of Treatment* supra
12 In re T *Adult: Refusal of Treatment* supra
13 In re J (a Minor) *Wardship: Medical Treatment* supra
14 *Airedale NHS Trust v Bland* (1993) 2WLR 316-400
15 *Frenchay Health Care NHS Trust v S* (1994) NLJ 268
16 per Goff LJ in *Airedale NHS Trust v Bland* (1993) 2WLR 367
17 In re J (a Minor) *Wardship: Medical Treatment* supra
18 Prof Glanville Williams, *Textbook of Criminal Law*
19 *Airedale NHS Trust v Bland* (1993) 2WLR 369
20 per Goff LJ in *Airedale NHS Trust v Bland* (1993) 2WLR 371
21 *Airedale NHS Trust v Bland* (1993) 2WLR 380
22 *Frenchay Health Care NHS Trust v S* supra
24 *Report of the Select Committee on Medical Ethics* HMSO
25 In re T *Adult : Refusal of Treatment* (1992) 3WLR 799; *Airedale NHS Trust v Bland* (1993) 2WLR 316

Euthanasia: the Dutch Political Perspective

Leonard J van der Hout

Euthanasia is a topic which, in the Netherlands at least, has occupied our minds for the past twenty years.

A year ago, the Minister of Education stated that a certain percentage of the lectures in Dutch universities would have to be delivered in English. The Italian press immediately stated that 'the Dutch language is being abandoned', and the Italian-Dutch Cultural Association reacted furiously. The facts, however, were very different from the reports. Similarly, decisions about euthanasia have caused a lot of concern and outcry in many places (including Spain and the Vatican as well as Great Britain).

I propose to discuss three areas:
     1 The definition of euthanasia;
     2 Facts and figures; and
     3 Political decision-making in the Netherlands.

Euthanasia as a concept has a long history, and the nature of its meaning has changed over time. It is a concept with a clear social extensibility, which means that it contains its own topicality and its own use and misuse in successive periods of time. In classical antiquity it meant fast and painless death or, occasionally, dignified and noble dying. Physicians were not part of this. Death had not yet been medicalised.

Indeed, it had not yet become a habit to treat patients with a poor prognosis and many physicians would have considered such treatment ethically inadmissible. It was therefore interesting for me to discover that

Hippocrates, the 'father of medicine', taught his students two thousand five hundred years ago to provide no-one with a deadly medication, not even if requested by them to do so, nor even to offer advice of such a nature; but he also told them not to interfere with patients who could be assumed to be terminally ill. Interfering with dying patients would not do credit to the physician.

The definition of euthanasia

Definitions are important here – what, exactly, are we discussing? The following three definitions of euthanasia are important in illustrating the rest of this paper.

1973 definition:
To deliberately start a procedure which will shorten a person's life or deliberately omit procedures which will prolong the life of a terminally ill patient in his own interest.

Definition of the Health Council of 1982:
Procedures which are directed at deliberately terminating or shortening a person's life at his own request or in his interest, either actively or passively.

Definition of the Commission of State 1985:
To deliberately terminate life carried out by someone other than the person concerned, at his own request.

This last definition is the one we will use!

I would like to make one important point before going on. Many readers of this paper will have had professional experiences with patients where the problems of euthanasia have had to be confronted. I do not have such experiences. My contribution to the debate is based on secondary sources and aims to provide an insight into the problem from a more detached position reflecting the Dutch situation.

In the seventies, euthanasia became a social problem. In 1975 the well-known Dutch sociologist Van Heek published a small book on the euthanasia question, in which he indicated how euthanasia could become a social problem. He mentioned four causes:

1 The rise of medical power and the institutionalisation of health care.
2 Rapid ageing of the Dutch population, causing an increase in the frequency of chronic and painful diseases.
3 Cultural-historical developments such as emancipation, rise of the permissive society and the mass media, and deconfessionalisation.

4 Creation of the 'caring state' so attention could be paid to meta-physical matters such as the nature of death and dying.

It was against this background that the political debate started. But before discussing these specifics, I would like to give some facts and figures about Dutch euthanasia practice.

Facts and Figures

During the euthanasia debate there was no shortage of assessments and computations. However, the figures given by those in favour were often too low and those opposed gave numbers which were too high. Since 1990, findings have been published from studies which give more insight into euthanasia and assisted suicide in nursing homes by general practitioners. In 1991, the Remmelink Committee for the first time published accurate data about the practice of euthanasia in Holland.

In the Netherlands, around 150,000 people die each year. Since 1990 the annual number of euthanasia cases has been established at 2300. This is much lower than earlier estimates which varied between 5000 and 20,000 per year. Around 2000 of the euthanasia or assisted suicide cases are carried out by the general practitioner, and euthanasia is practised three times as often as assisted suicide. These numbers have been confirmed by other research (Van der Maas found 1900 cases of which 1550 were euthanasia and 350 were assisted suicide).

This means that one in every 25 deaths is a case of euthanasia or assisted suicide. In hospitals this ratio is 1:7.5 and in nursing homes 1:8. Most general practitioners (nearly 75%) have received requests for euthanasia or assisted suicide. In 40% of the cases, the request was actually complied with.

It appears that physicians who have their practice in the provinces of Northern Holland or in the large cities in the south, and who do not have strong religious ties, apply euthanasia more often than those in the southern provinces or in the countryside, where religious beliefs play a more important role. However, neither euthanasia nor assisted suicide occur as often as was previously (and long) believed both at home and abroad.

Euthanasia and assisted suicide occur mostly among people suffering from cancer, multiple sclerosis, amyotrophy lateral sclerosis and AIDS. They occur mainly among people under 75 years of age and there is no difference in frequency between men and women. In 40% of cases life expectancy of the patient is less than one week, with 10% having a life expectancy of more than three months. In 50% of cases it is between one week and 3 months. Research has also shown that in around 1000 cases per year, procedures to terminate life have been undertaken without any request from the patient ot this effect. Around 100 of these cases involve the general practitioner.

One final statistic: the Dutch Association for Voluntary Euthanasia was established in 1973 and membership in 1992 stood at 55,000.

The political background

At this point it would be useful to give an outline of the political spectrum in the Netherlands, which has been an important factor in the decision-making processes that took place. The Dutch political map is built up of many different parties, all characteristically based on the large 19th century ideologies. An additional, and important, distinction can be made between confessional and non-confessional parties.

The confessional parties are the Christian Democratics (CDA) and three small christian parties based on the more extreme protestant principles. The non-confessional parties consist of the Labour/Social Democrats, the Conservative Liberal Party, Groen Links (a junction of communist, pacifist, radical parties and independents) and D66, which is progressive liberal. The division between those in favour of and those opposed to liberalising the laws governing euthanasia reflects the split between the confessional and the non-confessional parties.

Between 1978 and 1994 The Netherlands was ruled by the following coalitions:

> 1978–1981: CDA/VVD
> 1981–1982: CDA/PvdA/D66
> 1982–1986: CDA/VVD
> 1986–1989: CDA/VVD
> 1990–1994: CDA/PvdA

I would like to begin with the situation in 1984. In that year an initiative bill was presented by MP Wessel-Tuinstra on behalf of D66. At that time the State Commission which had been instituted in 1982 had started work but had not yet reported.

The Wessel-Tuinstra bill proposed that those areas of the euthanasia debate on which a reasonable degree of consensus could be reached should be laid down in law. The aim was not to introduce an experimental law but to bring a controlled approach to the complex problem. The reactions in politics were predictable. The CDA resolutely rejected the idea that euthanasia and assisted suicide could contribute to the humanisation of the dying process. The right of self-determination, the basis for the Wessel-Tuinstra proposal, was only accepted by the CDA in terms of refusing medical treatment. The small Christian parties could not accept this basic viewpoint, and they too were very much against the bill. The Labour party, VVD, D66 and PPR subscribed to the proposal in global terms. During the discussion, the confessional parties referred to Christian principles reservedly: their main opposition seemed to be directed more towards the role of the government, their contention being that the government should protect life absolutely.

In August 1985 the State Commission report was published. The relationships between those in favour and those opposed remained as before. The confessional parties continually emphasised that admitting limited forms of euthanasia and assisted suicide would irrevocably lead to further tolerance. In the meantime, the Second Chamber was almost ready for plenary discussion. The government also became active in the debate.

On January 20th 1986, the Cabinet presented its viewpoint. The Cabinet was of the opinion that the time was not ripe to change the law, and they had several arguments to back this up. The administration of justice and public opinion had not yet been sufficiently crystallised, enlarging the scope of the law would lead to a shift in boundaries and there was a need for international orientation. However, these arguments were not supported by the current law, and a Cabinet majority wanted to change the law to reflect their views.

The Cabinet provided and argued for a specimen bill, the most important difference between this and the initiative bill being that life could only be terminated where patients were suffering unbearably and where there was a high likelihood that death was imminent. In the initiative bill, and also in the State Commission report, there was allowance for those who were suffering unbearably due to a disease or a handicap but who were probably not near death (emotional suffering was also considered as a factor).

The VVD was faced with having to make a difficult choice right before elections. Supporting the specimen bill would have given a considerable concession to the CDA. In the view of the CDA, the Cabinet had already extended the limits from passive euthanasia to active euthanasia for the group of people for whom death was imminent. In the debate which followed, the Prime Minister Ruud Lubbers stated that the Cabinet would not give its seal of approval to the Wessel-Tuinstra bill. The VVD climbed down and proposed implementing an extra 'care' stage. The coalition was saved.

Despite a very heated and venomous debate in the Second Chamber, initiated by the opposition, it was clear that the law would not be passed before the elections. After the elections, the CDA and the VVD agreed to a pact on the legislation. If it were to fail, then neither of them would oppose the legislation which was in agreement with the State Council Advice. The cruicial government agreement established that for non-agreed bills in the Second Chamber, the parties' actions would be 'directed primarily by the desirability of the continuation of the coalition'.

The threat surrounding the euthanasia issue appeared to decrease. The CDA had succeeded in ensuring that the Wessel-Tuinstra bill would almost certainly not be accepted. The election promise of the VVD that the legislation governing euthanasia would be widened to take into account the rights of the individual to self-determination was hardly heard again.

After the elections in 1986 a Cabinet consisting of Christian Democrats and Liberals was formed. After six months, the Second Chamber received a letter about euthanasia from the Cabinet. Its essence was that euthanasia would remain an indictable offence but prosecution would not follow if the procedures had been carefully carried out.

At the same time the Cabinet proposed two more recommendations, but they did not seem to be in much of a hurry. In December 1987, the Cabinet proposal was sent to the Second Chamber. During the ensuing discussion, only the CDA and the VVD appeared to be favourably disposed. The rest of the Second Chamber offered considerable criticism.

D66, the initiators of the bill, were particularly disappointed. They felt that it was inexplicable that after years of discussion so little had been done. In particular, the right for self-determination divided the coalition despite the fact that the VVD had accepted, two years earlier, that in any coalition with the CDA this bill would be the only one feasible. The Cabinet (and within it the CDA) had won. It seemed that legislation would follow soon but that was not the case. In May 1989, the Cabinet fell and the demissionair Cabinet decided to pass the problem on to the next government. The new Cabinet this time consisted of CDA and the Labour Party – two parties with opposing viewpoints about euthanasia.

However, in the Cabinet formation a solution to the problem appeared. First a committee was to be installed to study the extent of the practice of euthanasia. Although the Remmelink Committee had gathered interesting data, their research was considered to have been a political move. The need to quantify findings had not been felt earlier (indeed, the Minister of Justice had stated that he thought it unnecessary). It was a delaying tactic; and it is interesting to note that currently the VVD (at that time the opposition party) has returned once more to its own opinions and is very critical of the course of things.

In September 1991, the Remmelink Committee produced its report. In general, politicians, doctors and others were positive in their judgement of it. Shortly after this the Cabinet passed a definitive proposal. The CDA could be satisfied because the new law did not automatically exclude doctors from prosecution; and the Labour Party agreed to the proposal because doctors could be reasonably certain that they would not be prosecuted provided that they had followed the correct procedures. In 1992, the proposal was approved in the Second Chamber.

Early in 1994, it was discussed in the First Chamber as well. A few senators of both the CDA and the Labour Party voted against it, but eventually the majority appeared to agree with the proposal under discussion, and after its publication in the gazette, it became law. But although one might get the impression that this solved the euthanasia problem, this is only partly true. The euthanasia problem has only been partly solved because the definition under discussion is very limited: it concerns only the request of the patient. Two conclusions come to mind:

Firstly: how could political decision-making possibly be carried through into the now-approved act? During the entire process it has seemed inpossible for the non-confessional parties to reach unanimous agreement about the view that euthanasia should be legalised, and accept the political consequences of this. Again and again, governing power (or maybe loyalty towards the coalition partner, the CDA) appeared to be more important. At the same time, the CDA has exploited its middle-of-the-road position. Prime Minister Ruud Lubbers may be blamed for having taken up an incorrect stance by threatening not to countersign a possible different proposal but the Second Chamber has again allowed this to happen.

Meanwhile, elections for the Second Chamber took place on 3 May 1994, resulting in particular in substantial losses for the CDA whose representation dropped from 54 to 34 seats. For the first time since World War II there is the possibility of a coalition between the Labour Party, the VVD and D66. D66 has hinted that if such a cabinet is formed, it will open up the discussion of legislation concerning euthanasia. This would mean the re-opening of a chapter formerly concluded with a totally inadequate legal act, so that the law could be reformulated in accordance with the long-standing wishes of the population (i.e. the legalisation of euthanasia). It remains unclear how the political parties would wish to deal with the problems.

A second conclusion is that society is developing further and that politics are still not able to meet the needs of those concerned with the euthanasia problem. Especially the developments concerning those patients who are so-called incapable of will and incapable of judgement. Finally, recently, a psychiatrist who had assisted a healthy woman to her death who had previously indicated that she did not want to live any longer, was acquitted. The Public Prosecutor will be appealing to a higher court against this verdict.

Conclusions

The average age of the population of the Netherlands is rising. This results in an increase in chronic illnesses. The part of cancer as a contribution to mortality rates will increase in relative terms. Medical science will be provided with more possibilities for alleviating suffering and lengthening life. It will not be possible to ban death.

Medical science will have to be careful not to be a threat to the quality of life, not in the least for serious diseases and during the last stage of life. Of all deaths, 30% are unexpected and sudden. In all other cases, the provision of care is playing an increasing role. Providers of care have to make decisions which are directed at, or are the result of, shortening life, or should one say not lengthening life. These decisions require a high level of expertise, capability and integrity. I therefore feel that this matter should be extensively represented in the educational programs for care providers and that it should receive attention in higher education. It is in that light that I see this symposium, one more step forward, made by us all.

References

Blad JR, *Tussen lots – en zelfbeschikking, de stand van het beleid ten aanzien van euthanasie in ziekenhuizen en verpleeghuizen in Nederland* Gouda Quint BV, Arnhem, 1990.

Boon L (ed), *Ethiek, Recht en Zorg, Dilemma's bij euthanasie, AIDS, begin van leven en grenzen van zorg* Stichting Sympoz, Amstelveen 1986.

Drion H, *Het zelfgewilde einde van oude mensen* Balans, Amsterdam 1992.

Heek F van, *Actieve Euthanasie als sociologisch probleem* Boom, Meppel 1975.

Hilhorst HWA, *Euthanasie in het Ziekenhuis, de zachte dood bij ziekenhuispatiënten* De Tijdstroom, Lochum 1983.

Hoogerkamp G, *Euthanasie op het Binnenhof: de euthanasie discussie in politiek historisch perspectief (1978–1991)* Utrechtse Historische Cahiers, 13 (1992) 1. Utrecht.

Jacobs E (ed), *De Bio-maatschappij, Rapport van de Vlaams-Nederlandse Commissie Bio-ethiek* ACCO Academische Uitgeverij, Amersfoort 1990.

Meerman D, *Goed doen door dood te maken, Een analyse van de morele argumentatie in vijf maatschappelijke debatten over euthanasie tussen 1870 en 1940 in Engeland en Duitsland* Kok Kampen, 1991.

Veenhoven R, Hentenaar F, *Nederlanders over abortus, meningen over beëindiging van leven bij abortus, euthanasie, oorlogsvoering en bestraffing* Stimezo-onderzoek 75-3, Den Haag 1975.

Vragen om de Dood Werkgroep Euthanasie van het katholiek Studiecentrum, Ambo, Baarn 1983.

Wal G van der, *Euthanasie en hulp bij zelfdoding door Huisartsen* Wyt Uitgeefgroep, Rotterdam 1992.

Euthanasia and the Law in the Netherlands

Gusta van den Bogaard

The only certainty in life is the knowledge that one day we will die. It is not death itself that is so frightening to most of us, but the fact that we do not know what lies in store for us: a long and painful sick-bed, mental impairment and decay. For centuries, people have tried to orchestrate not only their own death but also that of their nearest relations in order to effect where possible a good, mild death or a courageous, dignified one.

The art of dying, the 'ars moriendi' was highly appreciated in classical antiquity and the term 'euthanasia' is a classical Greek word which literally means 'a good or soft death'. The word therefore had originally no legal and/or medical meaning but a philosophical one.

There is still a considerable amount of confusion about the meaning of the term euthanasia: every possible procedure related to the ending of the life of a human being or the counselling of the dying process is placed in the category of 'euthanasia'. This results in many misconceptions in the discussion. In the Netherlands, agreement on the definition of the term 'euthanasia' was reached at the beginning of the nineteen-eighties, initially in the scientific literature. It is defined as: 'the deliberate termination of a person's life at his or her request by another person'. In simple terms, it is intentionally ending someone's life on his own request. The death of a person is the direct result of such a procedure.

In the Netherlands, the term 'voluntary euthanasia' is therefore a tautology, and 'involuntary euthanasia' a contradiction in terms. The request for a procedure to put an end to a person's life is an essential part of the definition. In the absence of an explicit request, there can be no question of euthanasia – but perhaps even one of involuntary termination of life.

The Dutch definition is a limited one. It is restricted to the description of the offence in the penal code, article 293. It is also a value free definition because it doesn't rely on conditions like unbearable suffering or terminal state. The moral neutrality of the definition is intended to eliminate confusion, by distinguishing euthanasia from various other medical decisions concerning the end of life. These include:

– *Firstly*, stopping or refraining from medical treatment which is in itself useful, at the explicit request of the patient. By constitutional law, a patient has the right to refuse treatment or to have treatment discontinued. The physician is not even allowed to treat the patient without the patient's permission. In this case this patient will die, sooner or later, as a result of the illness, through his own choice. It does not involve any question of deprivation of life.

– *Secondly*, stopping or refraining from medical treatment because it is pointless according to the prevailing medical insight. The confusing term 'passive euthanasia' was, and still is, being used for this medical decision: euthanasia not as a result of acting but of omitting to act. However, this is not euthanasia according to the definition. The physician does not intend to terminate the life of the patient by stopping the treatment or failing to initiate it; he discontinues the treatment because it does not serve a concrete treatment objective according to professional medical insight, and is therefore no longer indicated. On the contrary, continuing treatment against better judgement generally leads to an extension of suffering, prolongation of the dying process and can be considered unprofessional conduct or malpractice.

To be allowed to discontinue a medically pointless treatment, a request from the patient is not required. It is a decision based on medical knowledge, skills and experience which in most cases, will be discussed with the patient.

– *Thirdly*, the carrying out of medical procedures (including the administration of medication in adequate doses) which are necessary and appropriate by nature to alleviate serious suffering and pain, even if this has the effect of accelerating the patient's death. It is at this point that the infamous term 'indirect euthanasia' appears, but there is no question of euthanasia, the patient desires treatment for pain, not termination of life.

Additionally, proper pain management is an essential part of medical treatment and nursing support. The possibility of hastening death, owing to the use of opiates, is a side-effect of pain management which is not a prime objective but may be accepted as a normal risk factor. Often it is seen as a not unwelcome side-effect in the final stage of life.

Only when, under the disguise of pain management, the objective of the treatment is in fact the accelerated death of the patient, and an overdose is the means for achieving this aim, is it a question of euthanasia, provided that the patient has explicitly requested termination of his life. If the patient has not made such a request, these cases are classified as termination of life: uninvited and perhaps even undesired.

– *Fourthly*, assisting in suicide can not be considered euthanasia. Suicide means killing oneself, possibly with the help of someone else. The essence of euthanasia is that the terminating procedure is carried out by another person, and at the request of the person wishing to die.

– *Finally*, the decision to terminate someone's life without an explicit request to do so is never called euthanasia but termination of life, because the conscious and freely made request of the person is absent. In consequence, we never speak of euthanasia in cases concerning the termination of the life of those who are incapable of expressing their will, such as the mentally handicapped, the demented elderly, patients in a persistent vegetative state or children below a certain age, including seriously congenitally handicapped babies.

However, termination of the life of incompetents – an extremely delicate issue – is often classed as euthanasia, sometimes out of ignorance but also sometimes through bad faith by those opposed to euthanasia. This results in confusion and the whole concept becoming obscure. Briefly, only the deliberate termination of the life of a person on his or her request constitutes euthanasia.

Is this form of aid in dying permitted by law in The Netherlands? No; under Article 293 of the Dutch Penal Code, euthanasia is still a criminal offence. This answer will probably surprise you, since The Netherlands are often depicted in the foreign press as the Mecca or the Sodom of euthanasia practice, depending on your viewpoint. But up to the present this article 293 in our penal code has *not* been changed.

This discrepancy between the formal prohibition in penal law and the acceptance of euthanasia in practice, – if strict conditions are met – is possible on the basis of the judicial doctrine of penal exemption grounds. It can happen that the behaviour of a person falls completely under the contents of a penal provision and yet the person will not be convicted since, either the perpetrator appears not to be indictable, due to very personal circumstances (for example an absence of any form of guilt) or because the fact itself, all evidence in the case having been considered, does not provide an indictable offence: there appears to be justification ground for the conduct.

Since 1973 – the year of the euthanasia trial in Leeuwarden –cases of termination of life on request have been taken to court at regular intervals. Based on the ensuing sentences, the permanent jurisprudence has come into being that euthanasia can be allowed under certain circumstances and under certain strict conditions. These conditions encompass a hopeless emergency situation during a serious illness with unbearable suffering, that can not be solved by any other means which causes 'necessity or force majeure'. This justification ground was acknowledged by our highest court of law for the first time in 1984.

'Force majeure' means the situation in which a person becomes involved in a conflict of duties because he is, as it were, forced to infringe the law to serve an interest that outweighs committing a criminal offence.The circumstances which cases of termination of life on request have to meet in order not to be indictable have been laid down in case law too. These circumstances concern the decision of the patient, his situation and the manner in which care is provided:
- The decision of the patient must be well-considered, conscious, persistent and freely made.
- The illness must be incurable, and must involve serious suffering which is experienced by the patient as unbearable and for which no other solution acceptable to the patient is available.
- Procedures for the termination of life may only take place as a part of medical treatment by the physician concerned, taking into account the rules of careful medical practice, part of which must include consulting a colleague.

Apart from these conditions developed in jurisprudence, Dutch law requires that physicians report the cause of death to the Central Bureau of Statistics, and only the fact of the death has to be reported to the local records office with a death certificate.

Since euthanasia is not regarded as a natural cause of death, the medical attendant is not allowed to issue a death certificate but the local coroner and the public prosecutor both have to be informed. Because many physicians felt that they were unjustly being treated as criminals and were exposed to the possibility of a police investigation, they often covered up the true facts and wrote a certificate of death in cases of euthanasia.

In November 1990, the DMA and the Ministry of Justice agreed on a less consequential reporting procedure. After receiving a complete written account from the doctor, the medical examiner reports to the district attorney, who will issue a certificate of no objection to burial or cremation if he is convinced that the criteria laid down by the courts and the points for attention of the reporting procedure have been observed. If this is the case, there will be no further investigation.

However influential jurisprudence may be,
- court decisions are determined by the particular facts of the case and they do not change the law,
- the notification procedure was, until recently, a 'gentleman's agreement', and equally
- it is not the task of the judiciary to develop uniform standards for the required 'proper medical procedure and the careful decision-making'.

Our society wanted more legal security and it was felt that only proper statutory regulations could offer this. After years of attempting to achieve legislation – as explained in the previous paper – a bill was finally passed in February 1992 after a round of political horse-trading. The law shows all the signs of this and, according to eminent lawyers in the fields of health and penal law, it is a judicial monstrosity.

The new government proposal, accepted by the Second Chamber of our Parliament, is a sort of indirect legislation for euthanasia, and a very inconsistent one: The penal law will not be amended: termination of life on explicit request will remain just as indictable as before. Neither are *any* exceptions made in cases where physicians have acted with care in providing help, in accordance with the restrictions elaborated in the jurisprudence.

If prosecuted, an appeal of *force majeure* is still the only means possible of preventing a conviction. On the other hand the notification procedure is given a formal legal status by including it in Article 10 of the Burial Act and regulating it in a general administrative order.

The requirements of careful medical practice are, however, not legally established, but are only formulated as points of attention in the reporting procedure. By providing the reporting procedure for cases of euthanasia with a legal basis, a rather bizarre judicial construction has been created: euthanasia is a penal offence for the physician too.

An appeal of *force majeure* is the only means of preventing a conviction; but modification of the Burial Act implies that the same doctor will not be prosecuted at all if he commits the crime carefully, by reporting it properly in accordance with the procedure.

A far more serious matter is the fact that the bill declares that the reporting procedure is applicable to those cases of termination of life where there is no question of an explicit request of the patient. In so doing, the government is creating the impression that unsolicited termination of life is regarded as having the same status as euthanasia. By implicitly accepting euthanasia – by legalizing the reporting procedure – the government is creating the misconception that unsolicited termination of life can be accepted without any form of judicial control. After all, the reporting procedure which places physicians above prosecution applies here too.

All of the groups of Dutch society who have been involved in the issue are, however, of the opinion that euthanasia and the unsolicited termination of life are two separate matters. Termination of life without request must not be regulated by law. Grounds of justification exist only in exceptional cases, which can only be determined by judicial procedure case by case.

However, a large degree of consensus exists regarding the admissibility of euthanasia due to the crucial role of the principle of self-determination. Qualitatively good and consistent legislation was a very real possibility. Two excellent bills have been prepared, with the help of knowledgeable and expert lawyers and physicians. But as a consequence of the political self-interest of the Christian Democratic Party, something known in judicial terms as an 'obscure libel' is inflicting damage to a question which touches the core of our society's moral standards.

Euthanasia: an Ethical Approach

Frank A Huser

Our revels now are ended. These our actors,
As I foretold you, were all spirits, and
Are melted into air, into thin air:
And, like the baseless fabric of this vision,
The cloud-capp'd towers, the gorgeous palaces,
The solemn temples, the great globe itself,
Yea, all which it inherit, shall dissolve,
And, like this insubstantial pageant faded,
Leave not a rack behind. We are such stuff
As dreams are made on; and our little life
Is rounded with a sleep.
— The Tempest, Act IV, Scene 1

Introduction

The most important metaphor for the body today is the machine. The bodymachine has to obey the master's commands perfectly – ever alert, never failing, never tired, capable of lust and achievement. Above all, it has to be beautiful: no wrinkles, a perfect set of teeth and a tanned skin. Health institutes surround the modern person's life. Research in Holland has shown that health scores is high on the priority list of the modern man. Health as the ultimate happiness!

The image of the body as a machine has been described by the French philosopher and historian Michel Foucault. In his Introduction to History of sexuality, he writes:

'In concrete terms, the power over life has developed since the seventeenth century into two main forms: one concerned the body as a machine and was concerned with training the body, intensifying its capacities, making maximum use of its powers, fortifying its usefulness and docility equally and including it in effective and economical management systems; the anatomic politics of the human body.

The other, which originated around the middle of the eighteenth century, concerned the body as a species, the body which is imbued with the mechanics of the organic nature, and which functions as the bearer of biological processes: reproduction, birth and death, level of health, mean life span and long duration of life. They become the object of a whole series of interventions and regulating management mechanisms and are thus placed under management: the bio-politics of the population.'

This lengthy quotation goes some way to explaining the present-day movement in which health as the new morality, as highest moral good, has attained a place in our society. In the field of medical sociology, one hears the term 'the process of medicalisation'; behaviours and dimensions of life are defined in medical categories and come under the authority of doctors. Growing old is a disease. Few people realise that hardly anyone dies a natural death.

The new morality of health is a morality of fear; fear of disease and suffering, pain and dying. Sickness and death have replaced hell and purgatory as objects of horror and fear. We are constantly summoned to conversion. Modern medicine suffers from a Faustian delusion; ever being able to perfect life right through to its deepest structures, to ban disease and death and to found the empire of immortal health.

Clinical medicine is in a period of 'paradigmatic instability' the nineteenth century scientific way of thinking, characterized by concepts such as structure and function, has been perceived to be inadequate since the nineteen sixties. Rival theories have originated since then and are being slowly given form in epidemiology and the art of argumentation.

This development is the result of the introduction of new methods of research, the realization that the advances in medical technology will not necessarily lead to a decrease in the number of sick people, and the change in the biological-organic concept of disease into a more specific humane concept of sickness.

The change in the concept of sickness particularly is making medical science susceptible to philosophical and anthropological questions. Themes concerning the personal freedom to express one's will, the integrity of the human body (which is now relevant both morally and ethically as well as legally) and the autonomy of the person seeking help are gaining a steady hold in clinical practice. In both the field of medicine and the field of nursing, it is the patient's interests that are central.

Each doctor-patient relationship is morally qualified as a human relationship and evokes the question of what is good for each clinical procedure.

Ethics

The seemingly increasing need to view reality from an ethical point of view can be explained by the increasing number of possibilities for manipulation offered by modern science and technology.

Wherever human beings are able to change reality with the help of science and technology, they are constantly confronted with questions as to whether and how to use these possibilities. More freedom of choice generates more responsibility; in a situation where things do not simply happen but are decided by people, we have, by definition, to deal with the question of how to decide and how to act.

As the second explanation for this increasing interest in ethics, we have the increasing emancipation of the individual: we do not simply have a growing number of problems, but the individual perceives these problems to be his own as well. In other words: he cannot just go with the flow of his group, his environment, his church or religious community; he needs to know for himself why it is good or responsible to do something or not to do it. We want to form our own judgement about a particular event or phenomenon, even if we are not involved in it ourselves.

The number of publications in which the term ethics is defined is enormous. There are as many descriptions as there are publications. It is impossible to discuss the numerous variants at length within the framework of this lecture. I have therefore chosen a description of the term ethics which, in my opinion, is adequate. The word 'ethics' is derived from the Greek word ethos which may be translated as custom or manner. In Latin, ethos was translated into 'mos' (plural: mores) from which our word 'moral' is derived. Ethics and morality therefore originally had the same meaning: that which concerns the morality, the behavioral norm.

In the course of time, the word morality has increasingly acquired the meaning of an entity of behavioral rules, and the word ethics the meaning of reflection on these rules. This reflection may be aimed at validating the morality as well as the search for general principles from which behavioral rules may be derived so as to systematically reflect morality.

Ethics are a systematic reflection on norms and morality, the clarification of the concept of mankind which is expressed by them, and critical evaluation of this concept of mankind regarding its character of humanity.

Let us study this description in a little more detail. Three elements may be distinguished.

Systematic reflection

The starting point is formed by the description and analysis of the problem situation and the norms which play a role there, in regard to both existing rules and new rules formed as a consequence of the concrete situation at that moment. The first stage is vitally important. A systematic reflection aims in the first place to classify the problem. In simple terms, it concerns the question: What is it all about?

If a problem situation is described partially, incompletely or inaccurately, this will unavoidably influence the presentation of the question, which will result in the answer to the question being locked in a particular direction (by definition). Ethics is a science, a professional domain in which questions are classified with the help of theories. Ethics is not primarily concerned with our personal valuation, although that is also the subject of the systematisation. Ethics, in short, is not concerned with 'what you think about it'.

Concepts such as ethics and morality are often confused with each other. The concept of ethics is often associated with decency and respectability. In other cases, the term is used to refer to 'traditional', 'middle-class' and 'conservative' with an undertone of ethics which are 'not quite right'. Ethics may smell of narrowmindedness, interference, dogmatism, petty rules and 'knowing it all'. A nurse who lives by his or her conscience and helps a patient to relieve his suffering may be accused of murder. Such a nurse is accused of a lack of 'ethics', but this is quite unjust.

The difference in opinion about good and evil has to do with the morality and moral assumptions which are at stake. There is only anything wrong with 'ethics' when the decision-making process gets too tied up in caring, and if the argumentation is not logical or verifiable. Ethics should be practised as an independent discipline, independent of morality.

The concept of mankind

The second element in the description of the term ethics concerns the 'clarification of the concept of mankind'. Mankind asks questions about life. Mankind formulates answers to these questions on life.

Mankind is the only creature on earth which concerns itself with the philosophy of life. Who is this mankind? The answer to this question determines our concept of mankind. An enormous variety of such concepts exist and I do not propose to give you an extensive description of them and their origins. However, the fact that attention to these concepts is growing within nursing education and the Health Service is significant.

In the past, when people were admitted for the treatment of an ailment, they were predominantly regarded as physical objects, the sick part of which was in need of treatment. Now they are primarily regarded as human beings, as psychosomatic entities. The physical complaint is not presented in isolation, but is looked at together with the psycho-social factors related to the person asking for help.

Philosophy of life
I feel that it is important to take up the second element from the description of ethics, the concept of mankind, in a broader sense and I want to include the above-mentioned 'philosophy of life'. The philosophy of life may be described as an entity of symbols, ideas, values, norms and customs which the individual uses to give himself a place in the world and which give direction and meaning to his own life. This philosophy of life can also be found in the way in which people formulate their norms.

A norm has a double function. On the one hand it is the standard for evaluating our conduct, on the other hand it gives the guidelines for our conduct. At the same time, norms are always an expression of certain (true or supposed) values and the concept of mankind. In other words, there is a connection between the philosophy of life (the concept of mankind in the definition of ethics) and norms, or rather, the way in which we provide our norms with content.

This connection, I feel, is correlative by nature and is expressed in the last element of the definition: 'the critical evaluation of the concept of mankind regarding its character of humanity' (the most difficult stage of ethical reflection). At this stage, a reciprocal relationship between actual conduct and concept of mankind arises. The central question is aimed at the criteria for the judgement of the concept of mankind; in other words, on which grounds can the human be determined regarding the results of our choices and our conduct. The starting point is the fact of being human as an inevitable 'human being in the process of being formed', subject to many influences.

A body of ethics which aims to remain true to life will therefore have to be as dynamic as the human being itself is. It is therefore not possible to formulate the concrete contents of what is authentically human or ideally human in a sharply defined statistical concept. However, the demand for criteria for evaluation remains valid.

Dialectic process

In the description of the term ethics it was pointed out that in the third stage, interaction arises between the reflection on the concept of mankind and the actual norms.

This dialectic creates the possibility for continuous critical evaluation of what we are doing, leaves room for timely adjustment and prevents the fossilisation of previously gained insights. This interaction makes it clear to us that ethics cannot be seen in isolation from the culture in which we live. The dialectic process is an important fact. If we are aware of it, it will prevent us from making definitive statements and will guard us from attributing eternal value too easily to certain ethical norms.

The question arises then whether it can be said that dynamics exist in which no fixed points for orientation can be defined. In other words, is it possible to introduce certain fundamental basic principles when we are looking for human dignity? Some basic norms such as respect for life, honesty and loyalty may be suggested, but I doubt the importance of these ideas. The terms, although they conjure up a sense of authenticity, are to my mind too empty and too abstract and they will demand continual explanation. The possibility arises that they will lose any depth they possess.

I opt for a different approach with a more universal character. It is typical for humans to live together! Naturally, there are those who prefer a more isolated existence but they seem to be the exception to the rule. From birth to death, man is dependent on his fellow man. It is this experience which I feel offers a basis for determining the criteria by which human dignity can be evaluated. When people meet or, as Emmanuel Levinas stated so impressively, in the human face of the Other, the contrast experience takes place. Meeting another human being who shows his face to me is the first experience which helps to awaken my consciousness; it is a moral discovery which is at the same time the true foundation for a theoretical explanation of reality. I am concerned here with inclusive thinking, with well-understood self-interest whereby my own interest is only served, and may only be honoured, when the interests of the other person are not harmed.

Nursing profession

Within the nursing profession and in connection with the field of nursing, a clear development in the last decades can be seen. Theoretical development and professionalisation are characteristic themes, and here professional ethics plays an especially important role. The fact that a body of professional ethics exists, a code for professional procedures of a specific professional group, says something about the validity of the profession. Development in nursing theory shows the development of a nursing care concept alongside a medical concept, care next to cure. The emphasis is placed on the provision of care, particualrly in cases where cure seems impossible

This development in the concept of care has had consequences for thinking based on ethics. The high value of the development of the ethics of care reflects the fact that thinking about good and evil is no longer confined to rules or medical-technical principles, but is now aimed at the essence of care. It is not the application of ethical rules or theories that is important but the clarification of the moral span of daily care given by the care provider to the human being who needs this care. The ethical capacity of caring appeals to the care provider to use all his professional knowledge and skills to promote the well-being of people.

Well-being

The term *well-being* touches on the core of the ethics of care. We are no longer concerned solely with the physical and psychological aspects of human beings; the emotional elements are also visibly present. Attention, recognition, appreciation, compassion, gratitude and respect for the whole human being widen our horizon. This renewed reflection on our method of care surpasses the rule or principle and aims directly at its significance for our entire being. After all, that whole human being is the target of the care!

Life and death are inextricably connected. Death is part of our lives. The recognition of that within a wider perspective of care is the key to a body of ethics of care in which the total human being is of central importance. Respect for life does not exclude euthanasia. Respect for death may do so.

Ethics of care

How does questioning the meaning of suffering fit into ethics of care? Within some religions, suffering is regarded as having the effect of cleansing (some Christians subscribe to this thought). Such a view implies that people need to suffer or should not be afraid of suffering because it may include a hidden moral. In my opinion, suffering is only valuable when people take it on themselves voluntarily, not when it is imposed on them. Most suffering simply happens to us, and I am not convinced that this suffering has any value. In any case, we cannot determine for others whether their suffering is of any value to them.

Thus, based on the ethics of care, I classify euthanasia as a legitimate option which shows respect for life – respect for one's own life and respect for the lives of others.

> *We are such stuff*
> *As dreams are made on; and our little life*
> *Is rounded with a sleep.*

References

Beauchamp T L and Childress J F, *Principles of biomedical ethics* Oxford University Press, New York/Oxford 1983

Foucault M, *Naissance de la clinique: une archéologie du regard medical* Presses Universitaire de France, Paris 1963

Foucault M, *Histoire de la sexualité — La volonté de savoir* Editions Gallimard, Paris 1976

Rolies J, (ed) *De gezonde burger* SUN, Nijmegen 1988

Euthanasia as a Nursing Problem

Janny A Teule

In my work as a paediatric nurse, I was confronted with the following situation: a young woman, 18 years old, suffering from the terminal disease cystic fibrosis, asked me to help in terminating her life.

She had several pulmonary problems which were caused by her disease and she therefore spent much of her life in and out of hospital. These pulmonary problems caused serious breathing difficulties and recurring pulmonary bleeding. Antibiotics were prescribed but she had become resistant to these because of the great number of infections. In the end, these courses of treatment no longer had a rehabilitating effect. This was the pattern of her life: three weeks in hospital, one week at home, followed again by emergency admission to hospital. Because of her chronic illness, she had not been able to attend school for a number of years. She did not have many friends in her peer group and she spent much time in the company of her sister who suffered from the same disease.

The request for euthanasia was not initially put to the doctor but to the primary nurse. The patient did not use the word euthanasia, she simply put the main issue: she could not and did not want to live any longer. This was the start of a very intensive period of co-operation between the patient, her relatives, the nurse, the doctor and the hospital pastor.

After a lengthy series of discussions, it was decided that the request for euthanasia should be granted. The criteria for care were met: on a voluntary basis, a well-considered request, a lasting desire for death, and unacceptable suffering. As already stated, the co-operation was very intense and included numerous discussions.

The patient concerned indicated that she wanted to pass away slowly, and it was decided to administer morphine by infusion. In the end, this would lead to respiration depression, which would cause her to pass away. It also meant intensive terminal counselling for the patient and her relatives. After the patient had discussed her cremation extensively with her parents and her sister, they indicated that this was the time to start the infusion.

She passed away peacefully after one day. After her death, the entire process was discussed with the care providers concerned. This had been a very intensive process, an essential part of which was that the various disciplines co-operated closely and well.

Any nurse may be confronted with the request for euthanasia by a patient. This may occur either in an institute or in Public Health Care. However, little has been laid down as to the tasks, responsibilities and capacities of the nurse in these matters. Although it is the doctor who makes the final decision, the nurse may be actively involved as described in the case history. Because of the nurse's frequent contact with the patient, she will often be the first person to hear the request. It is assumed then that the nurse will pass on this request to the doctor. After that, it is a matter of conscience whether the nurse is in some way involved in the execution of such a request.

This involvement in the care for the patient who asks for euthanasia may lead to questions, doubts and emotional discussions and even conflicts. However, as stated previously, very little has been laid down concerning the role and responsibilities of the nurse in The Netherlands.

The Dutch Professional Association for Nurses, NU '91, has provided information for nurses concerning the euthanasia problem, which may be of help when establishing a viewpoint. In addition, the Dutch Royal Medical Association and the former professional association for nurses have provided guidelines for euthanasia. At this level, there appears to be agreement about the tasks, capacities and responsibilities of the doctors on the one hand and the nurses on the other.

These guidelines provide clear help. However, it is not clear to what extent nurses are aware of the guidelines. I would like to discuss the role of the nurse and the established guidelines concerning the euthanasia process. I have chosen to discuss these guidelines in particular because I think they provide a clear image of the responsibilities and tasks of the nurse in practice.

The process of euthanasia is divided into three stages: (1) recognition; (2) decision making; and (3) execution, or carrying out the process.

In general, the guidelines state the following.

- Each nurse is confronted with ethical dilemmas. In such a situation, she is professionally aware of the concept of life, norms and values which she uses when providing care.
- The nurse is aware that euthanasia is a matter of termination of life requested by a patient who is capable of making a decision, and that it is not a matter of terminating the life of a patient who is not capable of making a decision.
- The nurse is the coordinator of care and is aware of the medical, paramedical and nursing policy for each patient, and what the main aims and coordinating aims of the treatment are.

The first stage in the euthanasia process is *recognition*. Of all the providers of care, the nurse is often the most involved in the patient's life. Frequently, the nurse is the first person a patient talks things over with. As shown earlier, she may therefore be the first person to be confronted with the desire for euthanasia. Her contact with the patient is often very close. The request for help may be stated in many different ways, directly or indirectly. Euthanasia is a very difficult subject, which is not easily brought up. The patient will usually try to find out very cautiously how the nurse is likely to respond. The following guidelines concerning the tasks, capacities and responsibilities of nurses have been established:

- When there is a request for euthanasia, the nurse determines whether this is really a request for help from the patient himself.
- A nurse opposed to euthanasia on moral or religious grounds will inform the patient about her views when approached on this subject. She will take care that the patient has the opportunity to consult a nurse who does not have these moral or religious objections against euthanasia.
- The nurse who is confronted with the request for euthanasia informs the patient that she is not the right person to answer the question. She offers the patient the possibility of discussing the request with the doctor, after first receiving permission to do so.
- Nurses care for the patient who has requested euthanasia. In principle, the execution of the request is carried out by the doctor.

The second stage in the process is *decision making*. The aim of this stage is to analyse the request for help. This will ensure that a well-considered decision is made. Information provided by other disciplines is necessary to analyse the request properly. It is recommended that a multi-disciplinary team be appointed with the patient at its centre.

The nurse's task is to look after the patient's interests, to provide information about the non-medical situation of the patient and to test the care criteria already mentioned. The decision to actually carry out euthanasia lies ultimately in the hands of the doctor. It is important that the execution of the euthanasia is discussed carefully with those concerned at this stage.

The following guidelines concerning the tasks, capacities and responsibilities of nurses have been established.

- Nurses are aware of the euthanasia policy of the institute. Their task is to promote discussion on the subject if there is no such policy.
- Each nurse is aware that assisting in euthanasia is an indictable offence and that she may be prosecuted both by criminal and disciplinary law.
- A nurse caring for a patient who has opted for euthanasia makes use of both professional and personal arguments to decide whether she will assist in that process or not.
- The nurse who assists in the process of euthanasia convinces herself that all care criteria have been met.
- The nurse who is not convinced that all care criteria have been met will discuss this with the doctor and the nursing team, and if necessary with the management team, the board of directors or even the police.
- The nurse will inform the patient when necessary about the existence of the service for members of the Dutch Association for Voluntary Euthanasia and of the patient's right to choose his own doctor and care institute.

Finally, there is the *execution* stage. This stage encompasses the carrying out of agreements. Carrying out euthanasia is a medical skill. A nurse who has not been involved in the decision-making procedure cannot be involved in its execution. When the patient has passed away, both relatives and friends and care providers may feel the need to discuss what has happened. It is very important that the team meets again to evaluate the entire process.

These guidelines as established by the Dutch Association for Voluntary Euthanasia and the professional association may give you the impression that nursing involvement is of a detached nature. However, this involvement should not be underestimated. The entire proceedings surrounding the request for euthanasia is very emotional. The guidelines given may help the nurse in obtaining a clear image of what may be asked of her and where she may and can draw the line concerning her involvement.

As a final part of the procedure, I think it is very important that the experiences of nurses should be discussed. The after-care for the nurses concerned in this intensive form of terminal care is just as important as the after-care for relatives and friends.

Opposition, or towards a Continuum?

Frank A Huser

Salus aegroti suprema lex

'I'm not afraid of getting older, but what I fear most is the pain and the humiliation. I'm scared of the pain, scared in case I might not be able to cope, scared that I might scream. This kind of humiliation I find so inhuman; surely this can't be the aim of my life? Dragging on without any prospects, joy or meaning — I hope I will be spared this'

'I hope the doctor will listen to me, amd do what I really want. I hope they will let me say what I think is best for me. I'm happy as I'm living just now, and I want to be happy in death too.'

Although death is not a common topic of discussion, it is part of life, and there are many television programmes, newspaper articles and books about dying which make people aware of their own death. We are cared for from womb to tomb. We continually take measures to prevent disease and postpone death, or ask others to do this for us. Until the moment we die, our suffering seems to be entirely in our own hands. We want to be in control of our dying as well.

The discussion surrounding euthanasia often focuses on the doctor's role, paricularly when the perspective is medical, legal or political. However, when recovery has been ruled out the emphasis will be entirely on the care that is provided. What is the best possible way to care for people with incurable diseases? What is the nurse's role in this process?

Salus aegroti suprema lex: well-being is the highest good. But what does well-being mean for a person who is incurably ill? And who is to make the decisions? Are we allowed to end a life that is no longer a life, or, as a geneticist in the Netherlands wrote, can we end the bitter end? The question becomes even more disturbing when we ask: is it our duty to terminate a life which has become unbearable, when the patient asks us to do so. Care for the seriously and incurable ill is based on the the question of how we can support them. How can we surround them like a cloak which provides protection and support?

Sometimes the discussions surrounding euthanasia give rise to controversy. Ending someone's life, at their own request, is regarded as incompatible with the idea of offering care: 'care' in this context meaning the giving of support to a person who is dying. Palliative care, the giving of such support, is applied when people are incurably ill, and the aims of this kind of care are the prevention of unnecessary suffering and the combating of pain rather than the promotion of recovery. Although the shortening of the patient's life can be a side-effect of the means that are used, to combat pain for example, palliative care is not geared towards ending the patient's life. Euthanasia, however, is expressly distinguished from this. It has the aim of ending the patient's life intentionally, and at the patient's own request. Thus, the difference between palliative care and euthanasia is fundamental.

During the concluding discussion of the symposium, though, it became clear that care for the patient is at the heart of both palliative care and euthanasia. Both are clearly based on the concept of 'care'. We could therefore ask whether euthanasia and palliative care are really as incompatible as some people think. The application of euthanasia is not the same as simply 'pulling out the plug'. It is used only in situations where the patient, who is in unbearable pain and has no chance of recovery, requests that his life be ended.

There are profound differences of opinion about the question of whether a patient has the right to request that his life be ended, and about whether others are entitled to act upon this request. Irrespective of this, however, it is extremely important that we always have the patient's interest at heart. And having the patient's interest at heart is also the key principle of the care provided by nurses!

This puts the discussion about palliative care and euthanasia into a different light. After formulating accurate definitions of the different concepts, we can see that it is not so much the incompatibility of the concepts but the continuation of the care that should be the subject under discussion. When a patient realises he is in a caring environment, he may experience comfort in the parting from life.

Authors

Gusta van den Bogaard
Lecturer in Law for Health Care Professionals
Christelijke Hogeschool Windesheim

Susan A. Hodge
Lecturer in Law for Health Care Professionals
North East Surrey College of Technology

Leonard J. van der Hout
Lecturer in Sociology and Management for Health
 Care Professionals
Christelijke Hogeschool Windesheim

Frank A. Huser
Lecturer in Ethics for Health Care Professionals
Christelijke Hogeschool Windesheim

Elizabeth G. Jones
MacMillan Teacher
Kingston & St. Georges NHS College of Health
 Studies

Maureen McLellan
Lecturer in Palliative Care
Princess Alice Hospice, Esher

Janny A. Teule
Lecturer in Nursing Theories
Christelijke Hogeschool Windesheim

Janice Turner
Lecturer in Social Policy
North East Surrey College of Technology